I0397097

THINGS YOUR MOTHER NEVER TAUGHT YOU ABOUT GETTING OLDER

(A Must Read for Those in Their 40s and 50s)

BY

Suzy Nelson

Lavender Sand Dollar Productions

Lincoln City, Oregon

www.suzynelson.org

Things Your Mother Never Taught You About Getting Older. First Edition. Copyright 2014©. By Suzy Nelson. All rights reserved. Printed in the United States of America. No part of this book may be used or reproduced in any manner whatsoever without written consent from the author.

Copyright 2014©

Cover Art: Abra Damianna

Page Layout: Pioneer Printing Inc. Newport Oregon.

ISBN 978-1-5451-9701-1
U.S. $6.50

The intention of this book

I hope to enlighten people about the services available to seniors who need home care after surgery or other ailments. I am providing local information for the Central Oregon Coast but also a "heads up" to people across the United States to inquire about what their individual state and local government have to offer now that Obama Care and Medicare have been changed in 2014.

I learned by trial and error that my benefits differed a lot from 2013 to 2014. I wish I had been able to obtain this information for myself ahead of time but there wasn't any concise information available in a booklet for me to read.

I also am giving the reader a first-person view of my experiences in 2013 (Part 1 of this book) and 2014 (Part 2 of this book) as they differed a lot from each other in spite of the same surgeon doing a different shoulder replacement each year, and going to the same hospital each year. So, I learned that whatever worked in 2013 may not work in 2014.

The antidotes that I write about are something like those in the bestselling book, **Orange is the New Black** except my experiences have to do with medical issues and help recuperating while the other book is about a well-heeled lady going to prison for international drug dealing. She wasn't your average criminal but rather was more like you and I except she made a few very bad decisions.

My book is about you and I and the health issues and decisions that we will likely face as we get older.

It's great that we are living longer but it comes with a price tag—possible illness and the need for home health care.

Some seniors will opt for assisted living while others will opt to stay in their own homes as long as possible.

Whatever you decision about your future health, being an informed senior may make a big difference if you are faced with these challenges.

Author's Page

This is my fourth published book. My first book was **Andy, the Reincarnated Cat**, a children's short story about a red-headed man who dies, goes to Heaven and returns as a cat.

My second book was a novel entitled, **Before the Last Bell Rings.** The background of a gang high school is real but the story is fiction; a teacher with a horrible administrator accidentally kills her boss. What will happen next? Will she lose her job and her boyfriend?

My third book is a non-fiction memoir about raising my four preschool children alone in the sixties. There is humor and sorrow in this book entitled, **Now What?**

My Qualifications for Writing These Books:

- A Bachelor's Degree in English, A Designation in Public Relations from UCLA extension, a Master in Business Administration
- Many UCLA screen writing and novel writing classes

My books are on Amazon and I also sell my books personally giving the buyer my signature and a personal note from me.

Dedication

I am dedicating this book to my son, Brian Martens, because he helped me when I was in the hospital both times for replacing my two shoulders. He stayed with me the second time when we were told that I was going home the day after surgery. I would have been by myself in my two story house with my two dogs and two cats.

Brian extended his stay from my dismissal from the hospital on Friday until noon the following Sunday so he could help me to arrange for help at home.

This was priceless! I only have one son but he's special. Thank you Brian.

Table of Contents

Part 1 – Right Shoulder Replacement - 2013

When my surgeon, Dr. Brad Butler, asked me which shoulder I wanted to do first, I replied my right one, the dominant one. It hurt and the range of motion was very limited.

I was surprised that he could do anything to help it, let alone do surgery. I went to see him because my arthritis had spread to my arms so much that it was difficult for me to manage my everyday life.

I thought he would say that I just needed to learn to cope with it and then he would send me home

The day of my appointment I left two workers in my house finishing new laminate flooring installation. (I would normally not leave anyone in my house if I wasn't home but the trip to Portland, Oregon to see Dr. Butler took precedence over that.) I just knew he would tell me that arthritis can't be fixed but he didn't say that!

He said, in fact, that he could fix it. I was so excited that I called his office the following Monday morning to schedule the surgery that very week.

I hate pain and don't normally want surgery of any kind but this was an exception because my quality of life was less than optimal.

The only problem was that I didn't think about my being right handed and the handicap that would place on me for quite a while afterward for eating, dressing, driving, and many other tasks. I only wanted it to stop hurting and move like it was supposed to do.

It was tough afterwards but I know now that I made the right decision. My range of motion and ability to lift things with my right arm has improved amazingly.

I Went Undercover As A Real Patient

to investigate after surgery care locally in my Central Oregon Coastal area and Portland, Oregon.

These are facts as I lived them. Your experiences may differ with mine but I felt I needed to share my two years of life after surgery with you. (Two total shoulder replacements in two years.)

Part 1 is about my first surgery in 2013 for replacing my dominant right shoulder and **Part 2** is about replacing my left shoulder. While both surgeries were performed by the same Portland, Oregon surgeon, Dr. Butler, and the hospital was the same in both cases: Providence Saint Vincent in Portland, Oregon, that is the only thing that is similar to these two surgeries' recoveries except for physical therapy at **Lincoln City Physical Therapy** for two years. If you are over 55 and live in the United States, be aware that seniors are living longer than ever now which is a good thing but getting sick as we all live longer is a bad thing.

If you are very poor (on food stamps and Medicaid) you may luck out. Also if you are either very rich or have wonderful relatives and friends, you may not have to worry either. But if you don't fit into either of these categories, hang on to your hat because life will not be simple.

In 2013 Medicare and my insurance paid for the first 31 days of rehab after surgery which is a good thing. After that, a rehab facility will look at your insurance. If you don't have any but aren't totally poor, you better have a lot of friends and relatives waiting to take care of you.

In 2014 apparently the Medicare rules changed from the 2013 rules because they wouldn't pay for my stay at a rehab facility at all. I had to go home after one night in the hospital.

If you hire an agency (at least where I live), be prepared to pay $20 an hour with a minimum of two hours per occasion for any help at home whether it is for dressing, bathing, eating, house cleaning, laundry or pet care. That will add up quickly.

Your friends and relatives may say they will help you but

be aware—after the initial hellos are done, they will probably remember that they have a social life to tend to and be unhappy that you are so incapable of doing things for yourself, needing help for daily necessities.

Even generous payments may not prompt friends and relatives to continue to help you as they can't get inside your level of pain and inability to do simple, common things like eating, getting dressed, showering, and bathroom needs.

I had my right shoulder replaced in 2013. My left shoulder was replaced in 2014 because it was bad also. I have arthritis also in my legs and knees so as much as I wanted to go on with my life, my limbs were not working and prevented this from happening in a speedy way.

I was dependent on others for all of the previous reasons and also getting in and out of bed, doing laundry, cleaning house, and driving.

I am now able to walk around my house without a cane or walker but only recently (about three months after surgery #2) have I been able to drive for a limited amount of time.

Luckily mine is only a temporary problem but even so, it has been very difficult as my social life has consisted of my television, computer, IPad, books, my two dogs and two cats.

I have been going to physical therapy two to three times a week via the local dial-a-ride bus for the old and handicapped (which would be me). To use this bus you have to be able to get to the curb by yourself which sometimes is a challenge just by itself.

You can board either by climbing the steps or by using the elevated ramp (my choice). It's humbling to need to use this service but it helps a lot. Rosemary (pictured on the back cover) has been the local transit driver for 2014. She always has a smile and is very thoughtful which eases everyone's pain.

In 2014 I have missed going somewhere so this year I am getting help to go for water therapy exercise (my own idea) in a warm, therapy pool at our local community center. I may even pay for someone to accompany me to a couple of social events this summer so I don't go "batty". I need to have some social life in the good weather!

If you think this won't ever happen to you, this is a "heads up", a wake-up call. I thought that also as my general health is better than most for heart, lungs etc.

I'm glad that I spent 31 days at a rehab center in 2013. I had two therapists five days a week which enabled me to regain some of my strength in my right arm so I could remove the sling at six weeks.

In 2014 I was directed to go home after my operation and an overnight stay at the hospital. This was more difficult for my recovery which I will detail later.

I would recommend a rehab place with a good reputation for some of the time if you can financially afford it. While I missed my two cats and two dogs, my body was healing on the fast track in 2013 in rehab.

My house for both years has been somewhat in a mess because I've hired people to help me and I only have them briefly and often different people. I have spent many hours alone because the cost of help has been so expensive.

Bottom line—be prepared for isolated living without much social and medical assistance if you are home alone after surgery.

The good and the bad emotionally

It was a Sunday afternoon in 2013 when my son took me to the Rehab center in Portland, Oregon. I was heavily drugged because my operation had been only three days previous. I was definitely not "with it".

He bought me some basic things from the nearby grocery store and the ambulance shuttle delivered me in a wheelchair to my private room.

When my son brought the bag of assorted goodies he had bought for me, he gave me a hug and said he had to go home.

I cried just like a child attending kindergarten for the first time. I was drugged out of my mind and didn't understand where I was, no one responded to my bathroom call for help, and there was no one to talk to.

I couldn't even voice what the problem was but by the next day I had figured it out. I was scared, no I was panicked because there was nothing familiar and no friendly person to reassure me. I desperately wanted my family to be there to hug and reassure me that this was going to be okay. But, that wasn't the situation.

Prior to my son leaving, an administrator came in to my room insisting that I sign a Do Not Resuscitate Form (DNR). I told her to make a copy of the form I had carried with me but she insisted that I had to sign her form. (I was so drugged I couldn't understand what the form said but she was relentless saying I had to sign it so if I passed out they would know what to do with me.)

I ended up begging my son to advise me by reading the form because I wasn't able to do it. He did this. I signed it, and then he left.

The administrator lady finally came by and gave me a neck massage after my son left. That pacified me for the moment but I was still scared.

I did luck out with a private room and shared bathroom. I had a quiet room on the end of the wing with a view of the garden.

They didn't care that I had my computer, I-Pad, and cell

phone with me. In fact, they were very tolerant of my "toys".

The swing shift Certified Nurses Assistants (CNAs) even helped me when my computer went crazy and also advised me when the entire computer system was down for a day. This was a crisis for patients and employees alike because all the meds were on the same system.

Surprises in the Dining Room

When I was well enough and somewhat bored, Pat, my friend across the hall invited me to join her in the dining room for lunch so I could meet some of the other residents (patients).

I wheeled myself down to the lunchroom using my tiptoes to move my wheelchair. My friend signaled for me to join her at her table which I did but I wasn't prepared for the "down side" of the lunchroom.

Many people were more unfortunate than myself. Some appeared catatonic while others had trouble breathing or choking on their food. Many were unable to eat by themselves.

Oversize bibs were put on the residents but I protested politely suggesting that I would just cover my arm sling so when I attempted eating with my non-dominant left arm, the loose food wouldn't be too messy on my clothes.

As shocking as it was to see these poor souls, it did give me a jolt into the reality that I only had temporary limb problems while others had life threatening problems with many having multiple issues.

The food was gourmet and ample. While the serving sizes were small, it was okay to ask for more in the dining room. It was a bit more difficult to get additional servings if you ate in your room but I always asked for two coffees with milk for breakfast and dinner. They had to make extra trips to get that which I appreciated.

Some Entertainment

They had a daily schedule of activities that varied each day. For the most part, I did intensive therapy with two therapy people five days a week with long naps afterwards as I tired easily.

I put my therapy time as a number one priority but music was the exception. One morning they had a man play music on a keyboard piano—songs from the past.

He was indoors in the circular hub where all the wards came together. He probably chose those songs because so many residents had memory problems.

I enjoyed it very much but it did bring tears to my eyes recalling past events. A few of us sang along which was great. The poor souls who were nearly catatonic were present in body if not in mind.

Another time my bathroom roommate did an impromptu highbrow music session as a viola instrumentalist in a string quartet. While they were only practicing for a future event, we had the pleasure of listening to symphony music. (Unfortunately only a few of us were physically able to appreciate it.)

I never realized how important music can be but living without it isn't good. It really lifted my spirits and the camaraderie of other residents was awesome.

A Different World

No appointments

Unlike the business world, the rehab place I went to didn't have appointments for therapists to see patients. They simply went to the individual patient's room and requested time to work with the person.

I was baffled by this because I often had two therapists at once—physical and occupational. Actually this was a good thing because with arthritis in my other arm and in both of my legs, getting around even in my private room was a challenge.

I am thankful that I was near the door where the therapists entered our building in the morning because they often would poke their heads in as they arrived. That way I was able to try to kind of schedule a mutual time to work with them even if it was only a notation on the whiteboard in my room. (I appreciated my two therapists. It was dynamite as I understand that good therapy is mandatory for shoulder replacements like mine.)

If you don't do the intensive, long-range therapy, don't expect the operation to be successful for range of motion and weight lifting.

Other Visitors

The therapists were not my only visitors. I also saw the lady doctor who wore a long, unconventional flowered Mumu. She was terrific. Even when my skin was irritated from wearing a sling, she brought in her skin specialist to advise me on treatment.

She said she was from a family of nurses but nursing wasn't her thing as she alluded to the caring quality required of nurses. This surprised and shocked me as she seemed very knowledgeable and aware of my health issues but perhaps she meant that she preferred to use her brain instead of holding someone's hand.

Even Other Visitors

From time to time I think I met all the staff members individually in my room from the lady in charge of the food to the social director with her daily activity sheet. In addition there was the laundry lady, the cleaning lady, the maintenance man, and the weekly beautician. They were all courteous and tapped at my door prior to entering.

However, after experiencing the night shift CNAs with their ghost-like, quiet, helpful ways moving slowly in the night, the day shift CNAs were like a bunch of birds entering the building chirping their entrance at about 7:00 in the morning.

Overhead lights were turned on, vacuuming started, vitals taken, and no rest for the wicked.

I had trouble with this because it was such a jolt from the night before when all was calm. I considered taking my pillow outdoors under a tree. I didn't do it but I really did think about it. I could have left a note on my pillow—gone fishing.

Other Entertainment

Sunday afternoon occasionally meant a movie time for us. One time was a western and another time was an animal movie. Both were fun and were accompanied by a treat of ice cream or popcorn.

I had a view of the garden from my room. Pretty flowers and grass were in my daily view.

One of the student nurses took me outside in my wheelchair and indulged me by taking pictures on my I-pad of the flowers.

Lonesome Me

I have to admit though even with all of this, I got lonesome for my life back home with my two dogs and two cats. I even missed my vehicles including my new van that I had scarcely driven.

When they told me I could stay for a total of two months in the rehab facility at a low cost to me with my insurance, I declined. I really didn't know how I would manage at home but I knew the time had come for me to try it.

Looking back at it, perhaps I was too hasty about leaving. After all I had three gourmet meals a day with snacks available in between, a television, a private room, CNAs looking after me 24 hours a day with a RN (Registered Nurse) on each of three shifts.

Little did I know that at home it would be quite different— no twenty-four- hour care, no gourmet meals, and no RN.

It was good to be in my home but I paid a price both financially and emotionally to be there.

At home

So when you are at home, will you be able to live peacefully with no problems? Probably not.

One way or another, you will need help at home. Even if you have a significant other, will this person be willing to be at your side no matter what your physical limitations might be?

It's not likely!

Unless your friend or mate is destined to be a caregiver, they will likely not be in the mood to spend twenty-four hours a day taking care of you. Even a saint would be pressed to the edge!

So what can you do? Perhaps do what I did. I had to hire help at home; I live alone so I didn't have a choice. How much help will you need? That depends on the kind of surgery you had, the time you spent in a rehab center, and how independent your personality and physical capabilities allow you to be.

For myself, I initially hired someone to get me to bed, spend the night, get me up in the morning, feed me a couple of simple meals a day including my morning coffee, help me to take a shower and assist me in daily living: laundry, washing dishes, and light housework. I paid a weekly amount rather than an hourly rate.

I did this for the first few weeks. Then I hired someone at $20 an hour with a minimum of two hours each time to do only what I couldn't do for myself. (Initially this was almost everything but later it was only heavy lifting, assisting me with washing and dressing and light housekeeping.) At this rate, I found that I was trying hard to do more chores myself to keep me from going to the poor house.

If you are on Medicaid, this may be paid for. Otherwise you will be doing the paying like I did. It adds up quickly so I only requested help on the basic things to exist. I tried to do the rest, or in the case of filing papers, I let the work go without doing it. My slogan was tomorrow will be okay, realizing that tomorrow wouldn't be any better than today.

Clean clothes were left in the drier; dirty dishes were on the drain boards.

In my case, I wasn't able to lift anything heavy. Then I could lift a maximum of two pounds and I couldn't get the food in my refrigerator if it was resting above my chest. (My range of motion was nearly non-existent.)

I was told that with my shoulder replacement I needed to work out in physical therapy intensely to regain my motion capability. It was tough and pain was part of the gain but I spent many hours afterwards cuddling with my twenty pound cat, Andy, recuperating and resting. I also took some Irish Whiskey which helped ease the pain or at least it helped me to ignore it.

Of course, it depends on the kind of surgery you have whether you will have a longer or shorter rehabilitation time. I understand that shoulders take the most physical therapy for a full recovery, even more than a knee replacement. Now they tell me!

My other secret is warm water for swimming, a shower initially and later a bath or relaxing in a hot tub. After three months I was able to swim across the warm therapy pool using the breast stroke or the side stroke. I could even do some finning on my back which was awesome. The Australian Crawl wasn't even a glimmer of hope at this moment in time. My arms couldn't get the range of motion to go over my head. Even thinking about it hurt.

I wanted to just live in the warm water because whenever I went back on the land I hurt all over again.

Was I supposed to be a mermaid? Perhaps my surgeon could replace my arthritic legs with a fish tail. I'll have to ask him.

Social Events Or The Lack Thereof

After two months of being mostly home bound, even a ride to therapy on the disabled bus sounded fun! If the driver extended the drive to pick up or let off a passenger, I reacted like a school child with a chance to see what's going on in my town. When I wasn't able to drive, I took the bus for disabled folks (dial a ride) which I booked far in advance or I took a taxi.

A taxi ride in my community isn't very expensive. I also read, watched a lot of television, and wrote.

The Chinook Winds Indian Casino is near my house but I can't get there with my walker going downhill alone because it doesn't grip the road well enough. I would take a serious tumble down the hill.

On Easter in 2014, I needed desperately to get out of the house so I got a cab ride to go for a fancy meal upstairs at the casino dining room. I wore my new, long, red jersey dress with a rope belt. I even got a compliment from the younger man on the taxi saying I looked pretty. It made my day!

I didn't have any caregivers that day so this was my first solo social field trip after my two months of recovery.

Last year, in 2013, I hired a caregiver to drive me in my car to a couple of parties which cost a lot but it was worth it. This year, if I am able, I will drive myself to parties or do like last year and get a ride with a caregiver. I know of at least two summer parties and although I am not a party animal, I need some events to look forward to.

Parties are another assignment that wins the vote from the caregivers for an easy assignment that qualifies for work. Of course, I belong to groups out of town requiring considerable driving time. It's a good job to get paid for. Naturally food and drinks are given freely to whoever accompanies me in true party fashion.

I hope to do a couple of weekend events this summer (2014) with my RV group. Both of my arms need to be able to lift and carry the food to the potluck meals. I miss seeing my friends.

I also spend time on the internet browsing the real estate

for Palm Desert, California where I hope to move to help the arthritis in my legs. They say warm air is good for arthritis. I believe this is true because I've spent many days in January there and I can move much better.

Part 2—Left Shoulder Replacement - 2014

Well, I've been through this before, I thought to myself so this should be easy. Well, it wasn't as easy as I thought it would be. First of all there wouldn't be a rehab facility this time which meant that I would come home the day after surgery.

They had said that I should prepare for this but I didn't. I still held out hopes that Medicare would allow me to go to a rehab facility like last year but I was mistaken.

My son, Brian, graciously offered to visit me in the hospital and then drive me home, a two hour drive from the hospital. He had a high profile vehicle that I had to get into. The problem was that I had no energy on this day after surgery plus I had my left arm in a big, padded sling which made it even more difficult to swing my non-petite body into the passenger seat. It took about twenty minutes for Brian, the lady from the hospital, and an ambulance driver to hoist me into the seat. Even that proved to be a problem as I was facing the wrong direction and unable to turn around. But their persistence paid off and I was finally in my seat facing forward.

As Brian started to drive he said that I needed to think about the long ride to my home and the large volume of water I had consumed prior to our departure from the hospital. If I needed to stop for a bathroom break, how would I get back in his vehicle?

This disturbed me so much that I fixated on locating a high curb next to a restaurant for easy access to the ground. When I finally spotted one, we stopped and I raced with my walker into the women's room at the café only stopping long enough to get directions.

I'm happy to say that getting back aboard this time after stopping at the restaurant was much easier!

After we got to my house

We both came to the realization that I needed help, a lot of it. Luckily, Brian stayed with me until Sunday afternoon. He called a local agency that I had hired previously to do housework for me. When the lady visited us that weekend, we set up a temporary schedule with a caregiver two hours in the morning and two hours at night enabling Brian to return home, a six hour drive. The caregiver initially prepared my meals, helped me to shower, dress, and undress, do my laundry and housecleaning. Then after a few weeks we included taking care of my two dogs and two cats to release my neighbor from doing so much for me.

What is Available for Seniors Recuperating from an Illness or Operation?

It depends. Your income, not your total wealth will play a part in this. If you are in the low income arena, Medicaid may pay for home care or nursing care in a rehab facility.

If you have long-term insurance that you bought in your younger days, that would probably pay for your health recovery. Pat yourself on the back for being in the minority to have looked ahead to your future.

But if your monthly income checks including social security, Medicare, and retirement accounts total a low amount, you may be eligible for other programs.

For example, in Oregon where I live, there is an additional program called Senior and Disability Services (the Oregon Home Care Commission). A case worker will come to your house to interview you to ask about your income versus expenses. He/she will also inquire about the physical help you need at home. It is done on a point system. If you qualify for the program they will tell you how many hours you qualify for each month (depending on your income and need for physical assistance).

The injured person becomes the boss conducting interviews, hiring the worker, and signing the worker's time sheet. If you have been on a lot of interviews, you will be able to do this one but if not, they have material to assist you to learn how to interview. You will find it interesting to find out about the caregiver's background because with the private agency, you don't choose who comes to work for you and you aren't allowed to see their background. The agency decides which person will work for you and the days and hours they will work.

The state caregivers have been investigated for criminal records. The case worker will send the individual needing help a list of potential caregivers. The injured person will then select local people to interview to work at their home. The injured person then becomes the boss: conducting interviews, choosing the caregiver and hours they mutually decide upon, and signing the worker's timesheet for the state to pay the worker. The state pays the caregiver a given amount for each hour worked, often a greater dollar amount than the private agency pays the worker.

The additional bonus of this system is that you can hire who you want from the list and you can mutually decide the days and hours they will work, and request that individual to be the person to come each time to your house putting you in charge of who and when you need your caregiver.

Due to the financial qualification, not everyone will qualify for the state program, but if you are eligible, it's a good thing.

With the private agency where I live, the injured person pays (out of pocket) $20 an hour with a minimum of two hours each time (unless you have insurance that covers this.) The agency then acts as the boss, selecting the caregiver, preparing the timesheet and issuing payment to the worker (having received the private payment previously from the injured person).

Unlike the state run program, the private agencies will not let you always keep the same caregiver 100 percent of the time.

Also with the private pay agency, if a caregiver cancels at the last minute or if your regular caregiver has personal time off, the agency will send somebody else to your house to help you. This is often a newbie that you will have to train from scratch for your individual needs.

Who knew? No one told me about this state run assistance program, not last year nor this year. Not the Portland, Oregon hospital where the surgeon works, not the surgeon, not the hospital in the community where I live, and not my own local general practitioner doctor who seems to be hip on everything.

Last year I was able to go to rehab for five weeks paid for by Medicare and my insurance. I even had a private room, phone, and a view of the garden with a shared bathroom.

But this year when I was sent home the day after surgery this State program would have been a godsend for me but no one told me about it.

If you qualify you can get **free** in-home care. That's right. I said **free!!!**

I got word of this after 2 ½ months at home for my second shoulder replacement. To qualify you need to have a physical need for services and your income needs to be less than your expenses regardless of your savings.

Due to the financial qualifications, not everyone will qualify for this state program, but if you are eligible, it's a good thing.

The Bus
(with a lift for disabled people like myself)

Perhaps you are like me—not usually a bus taker. You usually drive your own car. I am the same except for now. Thanks to arthritis in my legs (and knees) in addition to my arms, whatever agility I had formerly isn't there now. So, I swallowed my pride and decided to inquire about the Dial a Ride bus in my home town of Lincoln City, Oregon.

The cost is only $1.00 each time you board the bus. Even that amount is discounted if you buy a pass in advance if you will be a "frequent flyer" thus saving you some money. At this time the driver will sell you this pass on board the vehicle.

I was fortunate to have Transit driver, Rosemary, this year. She is a pleasant lady and a good driver. We have become friends because I board her bus three times a week to go to physical therapy. I am able to take my walker which helps a lot for my independent mobility.

I am especially stiff on cold, wet days but with my walker I can navigate from my deck to the lift (think elevator) to board the back of the bus where I quickly locate a seat.

Passengers need to make reservations ahead of time as this bus has a busy schedule. They recommend reserving a month in advance for medical appointments and around a week for other things you need to do.

This bus serves the elderly and the disabled in our community. It also "hooks up" with neighboring busses to take residents off the coast and into the valley.

Rosemary takes her job seriously as she assists me boarding the lift safely and strapping my walker and myself into our proper locations on the bus.

She always has a smile and kind words for everyone even on those days when she herself is "under the weather".

Local people can reach the transit system for a reservation by calling 541-265-4900.

RSVP Trans Med Program In Oregon

You can contact RSVP at 203 North Main Street in Toledo, Oregon 97391

Phone number 541-574-2684 or fax at 541-336-1510.

This is a program where people volunteer to drive senior and disabled people to medical and other non-medical appointments. You do need to contact them to fill out a form for your eligibility.

You will be answering questions about your mobility (use of a cane, wheelchair etc.) as well as needing portable oxygen etc.

You will give them an emergency contact name and number and answer a number of other questions about your health and your home (e.g. number and kinds of pets you have, smoking or nonsmoking, and gender of your volunteer that you prefer—male or female.)

I personally used this RSVP once myself when I wasn't able to arrange transportation to my physical therapy appointment. A lovely lady drove me there and also picked me up after I was done and took me home.

She refused payment but I did receive paperwork later requesting a small amount so that volunteers could be paid from this fund if they so desired.

This is just another option in your bag of tricks for surviving while unable to drive.

How Long Should It Take To Regain Your Health After An Operation?

It depends. I can only speak about my experiences for two total shoulder replacements. In my case, it took five months last year to fully recover for range of motion and being able to lift weights. Because I am writing this during the second session of recovery, I will have to estimate between four and five months again to get my full range of motion and weight lifting capabilities. But, I hear that a total shoulder replacement takes more time to recover than many other things do.

What am I doing to achieve these goals? Well, I've put myself on a rigid schedule of three times a week of intense physical therapy coupled with two or three times a week in a warm pool.

Sometimes I can do the backstroke in the water and other days I can scarcely move which drives me nuts. My body dictates how intense and how often I can work out.

I wish I had a crystal ball to tell me that the third trip to the pool will be in vain because my body doesn't want to do any more that week but unfortunately I just have to go and try it. If I can't swim the backstroke then perhaps I can walk and swing my arms. But, it isn't for me to say because my body is in charge.

I have had caregivers spend two hours going to the warm water therapy pool with me. They have the option of either entering the water with me or just watching. I don't care what they do as long as they help me to get in and out of the water and into the dressing room with the heavy door that I can't push open.

One caregiver that I have at present is happy for this assignment because she is losing weight as she accompanies me into the warm water. This is a bonus for both of us and an easy way to earn money while you are doing it.

I am diligent about this. One night the warm pool wasn't available due to a problem with the chemicals so I had to go in the regular swimming pool where the water was ten degrees cooler.

At first, my body froze but then it adapted and allowed me to even swim the backstroke back and forth.

So, I never know how much or how little my body can take (something like **Dancing With the Stars**) but I try to go at the max at whatever capacity my body will allow.

Years ago I wanted to be in the Olympics for swimming. Now I just hope I can swim to gain my ability to walk with my arthritis and move my arms as I want to.

Why Use Caregivers?

They are needed for obvious reasons to help with bathing, shampooing, toileting, cooking and cleaning, along with doing the laundry, making beds, and reminding patients about taking pills, shopping and running errands, and even animal care for pets.

They also give assistance for getting out of bed, rising up from a chair, dressing, brushing hair and putting barrettes in someone's hair.

But even more is the companionship for anyone living alone. It would be easy to become depressed especially for a long time in recovery such as mine.

If you are lucky enough to have the same caregiver all the time, they can anticipate your needs often before you know them yourself. This eases the burden of scheduling their tasks and allows time for conversing.

<u>Caregivers</u>

My caregivers who came to my home shared some similar characteristics such as: being friendly, eager to work, wanting more work hours, and wanting the opportunity to have regular clients within a short drive from their home.

In my own case, I tried to get "regulars" that I could count on, scheduling them at pretty much the same time on the same day, week after week. But on holidays and weekends, all bets were off. On one major holiday, most of the caregivers called in sick which meant a lot of first-time newbies were put on the job. I had to do a lot of training which is difficult.

Also, sometimes the schedule is changed by the agency at the last minute. It is difficult for me to print schedule changes. My printer is upstairs and the arthritis in my legs has prevented me from climbing the stairs in my own house. I have to ask my neighbor to print up the schedule but he can't do it if it changes constantly.

I need to have an up-to-date schedule at all times to know who is coming and when. I am lost without a program (schedule).

I am pleased that initially I had a couple of ladies to care for me when I could barely do anything for myself. We bonded instantly.

My son saw me in the hospital and drove me home the next day after the surgery. He was concerned with me living alone so he helped me to arrange care through an agency before he left for home. I thanked him for being there for me because I live alone with my two dogs and two cats and I needed lots of help.

I can't say enough about the numerous things that caregivers do for others: preparing meals, assisting in showering and dressing, putting dirty dishes in the dishwasher, feeding and watering the dogs and cats, washing clothes, making the bed, vacuuming and cleaning the floors and bathrooms. They do all of these things while conversing with the patient and keeping their spirits up.

Another fun thing that my caregivers do is to take me to the local therapy pool for water therapy in the warm water. The way this works is that the physical therapists move my arm where it doesn't want to go, much like shifting gears on a big truck. Then the next day I go to the pool to do my own version of water therapy which is like a vehicle lubrication to get my arm happy with this new increase in range of motion. This water therapy was my idea because I love to be in warm water.

The caregivers like this assignment because they get to drive my new car, get in the warm water, and get paid for it.

I did water therapy last year also which helped my right shoulder heal but months later I only needed help for housework. I was able to manage going to the pool by myself. The caregivers were disappointed that they were hired to do housework instead of going in the pool with me. Who could blame them?

Think Pink

I like to wear pink so I have had many tops and some nightgowns in pink but now I have even more things in pink. It seems that my caregivers didn't separate my laundry by color. They just put all the colors together probably initially white things with a red towel.

And guess what happened? You guessed it. Now almost everything I own is pink. I ordered some new sox and other clothes on the internet to be delivered soon. You better believe that I will be watching closely when these new blue and white sox need washing. I also have a pretty turquoise, velvet, long-sleeved shirt which I will personally wash whether by hand or in the machine.

As for my white underwear, oh my! I use powdered bleach and Woolite but you guessed it, my caregivers just put them in with my colored things.

I hang up my delicate items but I found a load of them in the drier yesterday—bad news! Perhaps my caregivers are working part time for the manufacturers of intimate garments. If so, they will be increasing sales soon on my undergarments because the heat destroys the elastic on the underwear.

I don't mean to belittle my caregivers because they are hard-working ladies but I wish they would ask me before they do some of these things. Answering a question or two would be so much better than having to buy new items.

My first weekend without my caregivers—neither in the morning nor the evening was a test. While I like being spoiled with someone making my meals and serving them prior to doing the dishes. I need to have some down time.

Even trying to write this book I was troubled by having people around most of the day meaning I didn't have any down time to think and write. I found myself getting snappy even though I was trying to go with the flow.

This is my castle and only the dogs and cats are allowed to fowl up my schedule!

Another lady had previously put my bathing suit in the drier.

The good news is that it was an old, stretched out suit that I had used only for my back yard spa. Had it been one of my good, expensive bathing suits, I think I would have done something desperate.

I had company today. My legs have been so much better the last week due to my swimming so I didn't think it would present a problem. Boy was I wrong! I sat on the couch before she arrived and it was all I could do to get up again. (Thanks arthritis!)

I had wanted to straighten up my living room and put things away but because I couldn't move, I had to ask my neighbor to help me.

That's what's strange—one day I'm lively and can do things and the next day, I can't move! It makes it hard to plan my life.

Neither Fish Nor Fowl

It has been nearly three months since my second operation on my left shoulder. I am thrilled to be able to move my left arm in a rather dynamic range of motion but I still can't lift heavy weights.

I can even walk better than before (in spite of arthritis in my legs and knees that are missing cartilage). I can brush my hair but I can't put a tie on it to pull it back. I can put on my left sock but I can't do my right one.

I can usually walk up my stairs once a day but sometimes I can't. (and my two cats live upstairs)

While I can drive, I still have great difficulty getting into my new Chrysler Town and Country van due to my short legs and arms that aren't strong enough. (I have to kinda pole vault into the driver's seat.)

I can sort of take a shower but need someone close by in case the floor is slippery and I lose my grip on the stationary pieces of chrome that I am holding on to.

Initially I couldn't put my underwear on and off so I wore shorty pajama pants with a loose elastic top and a camisole instead of a bra. But, I can do it now—put on and take off a regular bra and panties.

I can't color my hair as I used to do because I can't reach that far with my left arm. Even shampooing my hair is debatable because certain positions are too difficult in the shower in spite of having an extension on my shower.

Scratching my back was a huge problem in the beginning because I couldn't do it. Even with a grabber it was intensely difficult. (I had lots of itches initially but not pain. No one knew why.)

One night when I was itching and didn't have help, I used a writing pen. I thought the top was secure on it but I was wrong! The next day I saw what looked like gang writing on the back of my nightgown. Had I been sleepwalking with some gang boys? That gave me an insecure feeling.

No, I found the guilty pen and realized that I had only been violently scratching myself.

My social life has also come to a screeching halt. Up until now I have had caregivers for two hours in the morning and two hours at night seven days a week. I paid thousands of dollars for this care but because I wasn't driving, my social life was limited to the caregivers and Rosemary, the bus driver for the disabled (dial a ride) bus. (Their personalities enabled me to get over the lonesome feelings at least until now. Watching movies on television and using the internet to shop have kept my mind occupied.)

Today I really want to get out to socialize but I realize that my standing and walking ability is limited; it hasn't changed. Only my desire to connect with people other than caregivers and bus drivers has urged me to attend some social events on my own.

I would like to go to a group I belong to but I realize that it is on a steep hill and whether driving or walking, my body may not let me go there now.

So, for now my social life includes three times a week for grueling physical therapy to regain my range of motion and ability to lift heavy things. I also go to the community center for the warm therapy pool with a caregiver two or three times a week. I was even able to swim the backstroke. But, in this in between state of my health just because I could swim the backstroke one day doesn't mean that I can do it the next day also.

I am indeed neither fish nor fowl—not totally handicapped (thank goodness) and not entirely well and able to do everything I want to do.

Comparing Last Year's Recovery Part-Time In A Rehab Facility With This Year's Full Time Recovery At Home

When I was dismissed from the hospital having had an operation, there was a huge difference between the first operation and the second one. For the first operation on my right shoulder, per Medicare for 2013, I was required to stay in the hospital for three nights prior to my dismissal to a care facility. I was taken to the rehab place in a wheel chair in an ambulance type carrier.

This was a huge difference from the second operation on my left shoulder. I had to leave the hospital the next day following the operation to be sent directly home thanks to Medicare not paying for an extra care facility in 2014.

On this second operation, I was heavily medicated so I couldn't drive myself. I also had very little strength. When my son asked me to get into his high profile vehicle, I had great difficulty. My body was just limp having had an operation the day before.

He couldn't believe that I couldn't find the strength so he advised me to think positive. I tried that but my body still refused to budge.

It took three people to get me into his car: the hospital volunteer who had wheeled me to the front of the hospital, my son, and an ambulance driver who just happened to be there.

Even though I was embarrassed, there wasn't anything I could do. (Let this be a reminder to you to check in advance for the current rules of Medicare, your insurance, the hospital and surgeon's rules, along with state and local regulations about getting care after surgery.) **There is no such thing as being too prepared!**

I thought I had checked everything beforehand but obviously I had missed the Oregon State one that would provided hours of free care based on my income and expenses. This was after I had paid $20 an hour with a minimum of two hours twice a day for seven days a week for about 2 ½ months. You do the math! It might look nice on next year's taxes but not nearly as nice as it would be to have that money sitting in my bank account.

Besides the obvious financial consideration, let's talk about the help I got.

After the first operation in the care facility, there were CNAs working all shifts along with a registered nurse on each of three shifts which helped for pain and comfort but also just for a friendly face to comfort me.

At home, I spent many hours alone due to the huge expense of getting help. As a consequence, I got lonesome, had to go to the bathroom alone, couldn't bathe unless someone was with me, couldn't have all of my meals prepared for me as I had experienced the previous year in the rehab facility.

<u>Preparation</u> is the buzz word here. Plan ahead. The future is unknown. If you get sick as you age, you need to have prepared for this ahead of time. (You may say you won't get sick but I said that also!)

At least I had some savings I had to use but what if you don't have savings? Get smart ahead of time. Check your insurance, Medicare, and your bank account. Also check out your relatives, friends, and neighbors to see who might be able to help you. Trust me, it's pretty scary to be in such a situation and then try to find out what your possibilities might be.

In Summary, I'm glad I did the two shoulder replacements even with the long recovery time. I realize I still have arthritis concerns with my knees and legs but at seventy-five I'm glad my health overall is as good as it is.

I hope my experiences will help others to be prepared for the future.

My Thanks To The Following People:

Nolan Kellow	Physical Therapist (pictured on front cover)
Charlie Mina	Owner of Lincoln City Physical Therapy (He tolerated me for the greater part of two years)
Transit Driver, Rosemary	Who graciously posed for picture on back cover
Erin Lahti	Photographer extraordinaire who took the Therapy pictures
Denise Hodgkin	Photographer for swimming photo on back cover

Local References

HOME CARE:

ADEO**	**541 574 8660**
Aging Wisely With Heartfelt Hands**	**541 265 8530**

**Current rates are $20 an hour with two hour minimum each time for private agencies.

State Senior And Disability	**541 574 3743**

(Oregon Home Care Commission, Dept. Of Human Services)
This state-run agency will assign a case worker to see if you qualify based on your income and expenses and your physical needs. If you qualify you can get a set amount of free hours of in-home help a month.

Lincoln City Physical Therapy*	**541 994-6252**
Transit System (Dial A Ride)	**541 265-4900**

A lift will transport you from ground level into the bus. You will see me on the back cover using this service.

Smart people bought their long-term insurance when they were young, years ahead of when they would need it. That's a good idea because those that wait, like myself, are no longer eligible to buy it later when certain ailments are on the DON'T INSURE LIST.

*My recommendation for good results. I speak from my two years of experience.